YOUR KNOWLEDGE HAS VALUE

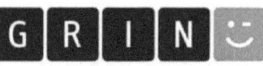
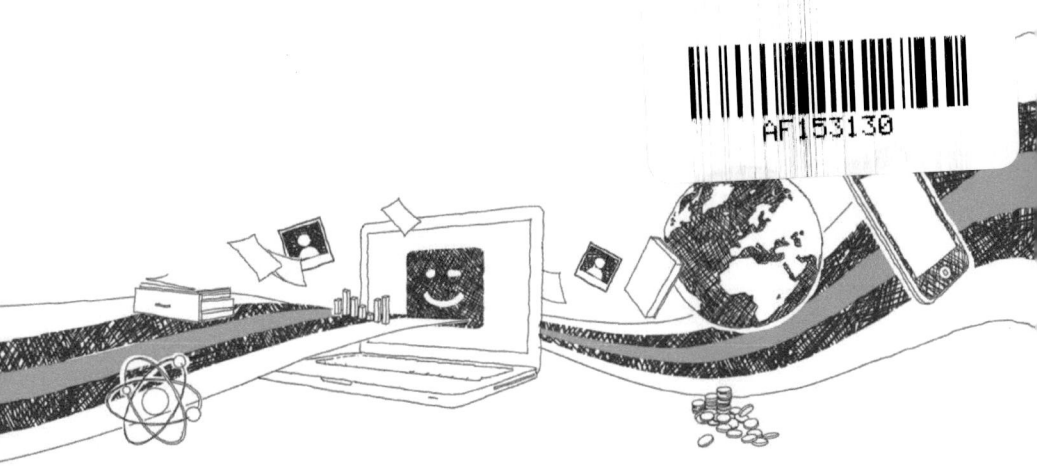

Bibliographic information published by the German National Library:

The German National Library lists this publication in the National Bibliography; detailed bibliographic data are available on the Internet at http://dnb.dnb.de .

Imprint:

Copyright © 2020 GRIN Verlag
Print and binding: Books on Demand GmbH, Norderstedt Germany
ISBN: 9783346123633

This book at GRIN:

https://www.grin.com/document/520670

Gizaw Mekonnen

Review on Bovine Schistosomiasis and its Current Status and Public Health Importance in Ethiopia

GRIN Verlag

GRIN - Your knowledge has value

Since its foundation in 1998, GRIN has specialized in publishing academic texts by students, college teachers and other academics as e-book and printed book. The website www.grin.com is an ideal platform for presenting term papers, final papers, scientific essays, dissertations and specialist books.

Visit us on the internet:

http://www.grin.com/

http://www.facebook.com/grincom

http://www.twitter.com/grin_com

REVIEW ON BOVINE SCHISTOSOMIASIS AND ITS CURRENT STATUS AND PUBLIC HEALTH IMPORTANCE IN ETHIOPIA

BY

GIZAW MEKONNEN

WOLAITA SODO UNIVERSITY
SCHOOL OF VETERINARY MEDICINE

APRIL, 2020

WOLAITA SODO, ETHIOPIA

TABLE OF CONTENT PAGE

LIST OF TABLES

LIST OF FIGURES

ABBREVIATIONS AND ACCRONYMS

DVM	Doctor of Veterinary medicine
NTD	Neglected Tropical Disease
WHO	World Health Organization
COPT	Circumoval Precipitin Test
IHA	Indirect Hemaglutination Assay
IWMI Inistitute	International Water Manegment
AAU	Addis Abeba University
DVM	Doctor of Veterinary Medicine
FVM	Faculty of Veterinary Medicine

SUMMARY

Schistosomiasis is a parasitic disease transmitted by snail intermediate hosts. It is one of the most wide spread zoonotic disease which is endemic in many developing countries of the tropics and sub tropics causing considerable loss in humans and animals. The disease affects rural communities particularly those who depend upon irrigation to support their agriculture. Currently it affects between 200 and 300 million people in around 74 countries. The great majority (80-85%) of schistosomiasis is found in sub-Saharan Africa. Schistosomiasis is caused by trematode worms of the genus Schistsoma that live in the alimentary tract, bladder, as well as hepatic and nasal veins of humans and animals.

Effective transmission of schistosomiasis occurs when the schistosome parasites, the aquatic snail hosts and the human or animal definitive hosts meet in space and time in surface water. The pathological changes with the disease are attributed by the adult parasite, cercaria and the eggs of the parasite. Health education, chemotherapy, environmental and biological control as well as provision of clean water have an innumerable role in the control activity of the disease. The use of traditional medicines in the treatment of schistosomiasis are economically important and a growing concern.

There are various types of plants having anti schistosomal and molluscicidal properties with minimal side effects used by developing countries and continuous to be used in the modern world. Phytoplacca dodecandora (Endod) is the most widely studied molluscicide in Ethiopia.

Key words: Endod, Medicinal Plants,Molluscicide, Schistosomiasis

INTRODUCTION

Schistosomiasis or bilharizia is one of the snail borne trematode infection of animals and humans caused by genus schistosoma and occurring in different parts of tropical and sub tropical countries. Unlike other trematodes, the schistosomes are dioecious , *i.e.,the sexes are separated.* The male surrounds the female and encloses her with in his *gynacophoric canal* for the entire adult lives of the worms. (*Samuel et al, 2016*). Schistosomiasis is a common parasitic infection of cattle mainly, in Africa and Asia, in which about 530 million heads of cattle live in areas endemic for cattle schistosomiasis and it has been reported that 165 million cattle becomes infected with Schistosomiasis all world wide. The passive immunity of the calves which they received by the colostrum in the prenatal and postnatal period reacts for the infection which they receive in the early age through water contact (Gabriel *et al*, 2002).

Ethiopia is highly endemic for Schistosomiasis, since temperature in Ethiopia appears to be the major factor that affects the distribution of Schistosoma species (WHO, 2010). Out of 10 species reported to naturally infected cattle, six have received particular attention mainly because of their recognized veterinary significance. The major species that cause animal schistosomiasis include: *Schistosoma bovis, S. indicum, S. japonicum, S. matthei, S. intercalatum, S. nasale* and *S.rodhoni* (Jejaw*et al.*, 2015). S. *bovis, S. matthei* and *S.intercalatum* are the most important species that can cause schistosomiasis in ruminants.

The geographical distribution of bovine schistosomiasis has been determined primarily by the distribution of snail intermediate host particularly *Bulinus* species which are important for the occurrence of disease in bovine species. *Schistosoma bovis* is a species' whose final hosts are bovines, ovines, caprines and whose secondary hosts are small wild ruminants.

They are distributed through out Africa, South West Asia and Mediterranean, Europe (Urquhart *et al.*, 2003).

The increasing use of irrigation in agriculture and fish breeding facilitate to increase number of snails which carry *Schistosoma* and as a consequence the human and animal incidence of schistosomiasis is increases. More over, level of infection, the frequency of water contacts and increasing cattle mobility through trading or rental increased the possibility of spreading the disease or infection sources (Islam *et al.*, 2011).

In human the disease is common in about 74 developing countries and mainly affects people living in rural agricultural and peri-urban areas (Oliveira, 2004). The principal clinical signs in the affected host are mainly associated with passage of the spindle eggs through the tissue of the gut lumen. The young parasites cause some damage during migration, but most of the lesions are due to the irritation produced by the eggs of the parasites in the intestine and other organs(Marquardt and Greive, 2000; Bowman *et al.*, 2003).

Diagnosis is primarily based on the clinico-pathological picture, seasonal occurrence, and previous history of schistosomiasis in the area or the identification of snail habitats with a history of access to natural water bodies. Praziquantel is highly effective for the treatment of bovine schistosomiasis. The goal of treatment is reduction of egg production via reduction of worm load: this reduces mortality and morbidity (Richer, 2003).

The most effective way to control cattle schistosomiasis in endemic areas is to prevent contact between the animals and the parasite. But this is not always practical in some parts of the world where nomadic conditions of management prevail, so that destruction of the snail intermediate host population at transmission sites, either by chemical or biological methods, or their removal by mechanical barriers or snail traps are some methods used as a control of the disease (Bont, 1995).

The objectives of this seminar paper is listed by the following way

- ➢ To review bovine schistosomiasis .
- ➢ To rechake the current status and public health siginifficance of bovine schistosomiasis in Ethiopia.

2. BOVINE SCHISTOSOMIASIS

2.1 Etiology

Schistosomiasis are caused by genus schistosoma.There are many species under the genus Schistosoma. However, the most important species both in human and veterinary field that causes pathological changes in their associated organs or predilection sites are S. nasale, S. bovis, S. indicum, S. spindale, S. hematobium, S. intercalatum, S. japonicum and S. mattheei (Mandal, 2006).

2.1.1 Morphology of Schistosoma
Adult schistosomes have a basic bilateral symmetry, oral and ventral suckers, a body covering of asyncytial tegument, a blind-ending digestive system consisting of mouth, esophagus and bifurcated tail Schistosomes exhibit sexual dimorphism and have distinct separate sexes. Adult worms are about 0.3-3 cm in length that lives in the blood vessels around the intestine, hepatic, nasal or bladder veins. The mature male worm is broad and flat, in wardly curved forming a groove called gynaecophoric canal to clap the female which is longer than the male (Lefevre,*et al* 2010). The female worm after copulation is set free to lay its eggs. Each mature female produces about two hundred ova per day.

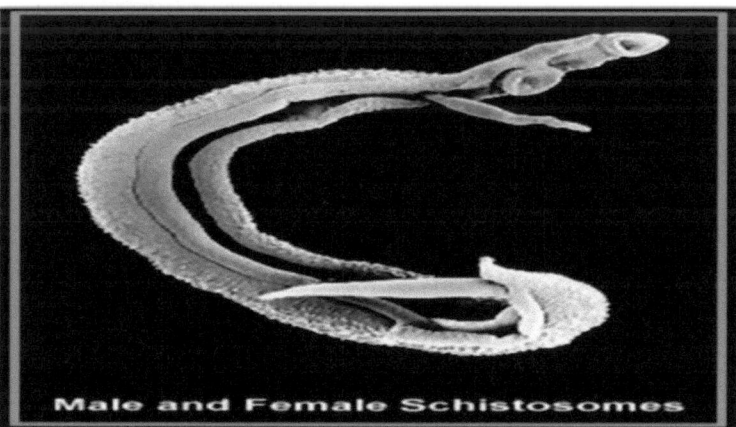

Figure 1: Mature schistosome worm: female lying in the gynaecophoric canal of male.
Source: springer 2001

3

2.1.2 Taxonomy

The taxonomic classification of the organism is presented as kingdom Animalia, Phylum Platyhelminthes, class Trematoda, sub class digenea,Family Schistosomatidae, Genus Schistosoma and species *Schistosoma bovis, Schistosoma leiperi, Schistosoma mattheei, Schistosoma mansoni, Schistosoma hematobium, Schistosoma nasalis, Schistosoma japonicum, Schistosoma spindale, Schistosoma indicum and Schistosoma Intercalatum*(Dwight *et al*, 2003).Schistosomiasis is a chronic debilitating parasitic disease of both human and animals, and is caused by different species of the genus Schistosoma (Pari-jia, 2004). Generally the eggs have typical morphological features. Relatively larger, slender (spindle) shaped and have lateral of terminal spine (pointed at both ends) (*Urquhart et al.*, 2003).

2.2 Epidemiology

High rain fall is good predisposing factor for the occurrence of the parasite(Mandal, 2006). Particularly it is common in tropical and subtropical countries like Africa, Caribbean, Southeastern America, East Asia and in the Middle East. The disease affects between 200and300 million people in around 74countries. Over 600 million people are reported to be at risk of this trematode disease (Ibrahim , 2009)..

The great majority (80-85%) of schistosomiasis is found in sub-Saharan Africa, due to low socioeconomy or favorable climate for breeding of the snail and transmission of the disease (Liang,*et al*, 2007). In Ethiopia, various epidemiological studies conducted on cattle schistosomiasis were indicative of the epidemicity of the disease in large stagnant water bodies and marshy free grazing areas. The prevalence of *S.bovis* has reported from different regions of the country by fecal examination (Mersha,*et al*,2012). About 29.89 million people are at risk of acquiring schistosomiasis and of these 4 million are infected. The incidence in Ethiopia is increased by construction of dams, expansion of irrigation based agriculture schemes and population movements.

The intermediate hosts having veterinary and public health importance belong to the genus *Biomphalaria*, *Bulinus*, Oncomelania, *Indoplanorbis*, *Planorbis* , *Radix* and there are about 350 species. Most of these snails are aquatic that live under the water and can not usually survive elsewhere. But there are also amphibious snails adapted for living in and out of water (*Oncomelania*). A large population of snails are live in fresh waters, where the larvae of genus *Biomphalaria* serve as intermediate hosts of parasitic trematodes also pass part of their life (Singh,*et al* 2000) .

Snail of the *S.mansoni* in Africa and America and *Bulinus* serve as the intermediate hosts of *S. haematobium* in Africa and the intermediate hosts of *S.haematobium* in Africa and the *Oncomelania* and *Tricula* serve as the intermediate hosts of *S.japonicum* and *S.mekongi,* respectively. Cattle, sheep, goat zebra, horse, pig, dog, donkey man, and birds are meracida recovery through culturing (Laikemariam,*et al*, 2005). In areas endemic for Schistosoma, detection of spindle shaped eggs having lateral or terminal spine depending on the the gold standard technique of Schistosomiasis diagnosis (Kassi, , 1999)..

It is almost similar to fasciola gigantica and paramphistomes. Schistosoma required water for hatching of the eggs. Eggs can hatch in slightly acidic ph. Sheding of cercariae is temperature dependent. Long time is required for development of shcistosoma in snail high rainfall is good predisposing factor for occurrence of these parasites (Mandal, 2012)

.Epidemiological studies on bovine schistosomiasis are suggestive of the endemicity of the disease particularly in areas with large permanent water bodies and marshy pasture areas. In Ethiopia, the optimum range for distribution of S.mansoni has been reported as 1500 to 2000 meter above sea level (masl) (Gashaw, 2010).Geographic distribution, natural hosts and anatomical site of Schistosoma species were illustrated in table 1

Table1.Definitive hosts, predilection site and geographic distribution of s. species.

Species	Natural definitive host	Anatomic site of adult fluke	Geographic Distribution
S. japonica	Human, dogs, cats rat, cattle, sheep, water buffalo, goat, horse, swine	Mesenteric and portal veins hemorrhoidal plexus	Chaina, Japan Taiwan, Celebes, Philippines.
S. haematobium	Humans, monkey	Pelvic veins and especially vesicle and mesenteric, vesicoprostatic, pubic and uterine plexus	Africa, western Asia, southern Europe Australia
S .mansion	Humans, monkey	Mesenteric and portal veins, hemorrhoid plexus	Africa, south America, India
S. bovid	Cattle, sheep, goat horse, mule, antelope, baboon	Portal and mesenteric veins	Africa, southern Asia, Sardinia
S. Spindale	Cattle, sheep, goat, antelope, water buffalo, doge	Mesenteric & portal veins	Africa, India
S. incognitum	Dog, pig	Mesenteric &portal veins	India
S. nasalis	Cattle, goats, horses	Nasal veins	India
S. indicum	Cattle, sheep, goats, horse, camels	Mesenteric, portal & pelvic veins	India
S. interculatum	Humans, horses, cattle, sheep,	Mesenteric &portalviens	Africa
S. mattheei	Cattle, sheep, goats, horse & rarely humans	Mesenteric & portal veins	Africa

Source: Jones *et al.* (1983)2.

2.2.1. Risk factors for infection

2.2.1.1. Host related risk factors

Age

This might be occured due to a long exposure time because older animals move long distances in search of scarce pastures and water thereby increasing their chances of infection as well as becoming infected at overcrowded watering holes. On the other hand, the very young calf do not graze extensively as the older, so they get less infection chance of cercariae unlike adult animals. Kassaw (2007) and (Nagiet al., 1999) also reported that the increased contact time with schistosoma infested habitat increases the rate and endemicity of schistosomiasis. Infection rate increased with the increase of age and peak infection occurred at the maturity of age (Bedarkaret al., 2000).

Sex

Differences in susceptibility to infection between sexes have been observed by various workers. The observed disparity may not solely due to difference in susceptibility but may also depend on a sex-related variation in behavior that results in differences in exposure (Magona and Musisi, 2002).

The reason seems to be related to social practice of keeping females under better management and feeding condition for milk production and Males are also fed relatively poor diet which increases the susceptibility to parasitic infection (Houdijk and Athana, 2003).

Breed

According to the (Alemsegedet al. 2010) reportes the local breeds are more affected by schistosomiasis than cross breeds. This difference in prevalence of the disease does not appear to be due to the difference in susceptibility but due to the difference in exposure. Cross breeds are mostly kept for dairy or fattening purpose and they are mostly housed and supplementing good feed and clean water which reduce their access to the cercariae.

7

However, the local once are mostly managed extensively to graze freely and get access to infective stage of the parasite.

Immunity

Cattle residing in endemic areas show a typical pattern in faecal egg counts. The faecal egg excretion usually starts between 4 and 8 months of life, counts increase rapidly to reach a maximum around the age of 6–15 months and then decrease markedly by the age of 18 months (De Bont and Vercruysse, 1997). In older animals, faecal egg counts remain low, tissue egg counts seem to follow the pattern of the faecal egg counts, while worm burden tends to increase with the age of the host (vercruysse& Gabriel, 2005).

The suppression in egg production is probably induced by serum-born factors, since adult worms from cattle with naturally acquired immunity to *S. bovi*s, surgically transplanted into non-immune animals, produced large number of eggs again (Bushura*et al.,* 1982, Bushura*et al.,* 1994). Reductions in worm burden and egg counts could also be induced in non-immune calves, which received serum from immune donors (Bushura*et al.,* 1994).

A few studies reported on heterologous resistance. Calves previously exposed to infection with the human schistosomes *S. mansoni* and *S. haematobium* were partially protected against *S. mattheei* and *S. bovis*, and it was believed that this type of heterologous resistance might be of considerable importance in protecting cattle from the more serious effects of schistosomiasis (De Bont and Vercruysse, 1997).

2.2.1.2. Seasonal risk factor

Schistosome infection rate in cattle increases during rainy season. The highest infection rate in rainy season could be due to abundance of snails and their rapid multiplication and dispersion.

Furthermore, dispersion of fecal matter occurs due to rain splashes. These factors may enhance the infection of snails by miracidia and cercarial contamination to adjacent areas through water. During this time conditions on the lands are suitable for the survival of the intermediate hosts and they become heavily infected with the schistosome larval stages. So, cattle are prone to get the infection of schistosomes (Soulsby, 1982). But in dry season infection rate of the schistosome parasite is low because of harsh dry conditions and less chances of infection due to unavailability of snail intermediate hosts as the water sources are scarce in this season (Kahn, 2011).

2.2.1.3. Management risk factors

This might be occured due to the lose of better management practices and sanitation Belayneh and Tadesse,(2014) highlighted the fact that proper management practices and policy change towards urban husbandry can minimize the schistosomiasis prevalence. They also reported that when cattle are slaughtered through back yard system and consequently the stomach and other intestinal contents including blood and washed materials are dumped into the nearby water bodies' prevalence of the disease also increases.

In the semi-intensive system of rearing where animals grazing in the fields have more risks of getting contact with water and subsequently with the infective stage, cercaria. Moreover, increasing cattle mobility through trading and   potentially increases the possibility of spreading the disease or infection sources (Kahn, 2011).

In addition to management risk factors, cattle schistosomiasis is dependent on environmental factors such as moisture, rain fall, temperature, presence of water bodies (stagnant, swampy, and marshy) and snail intermediate hosts.

Husbandry practice such as grazing system, keeping animals whether they are kept all together and / or separately, feeding (contaminated pasture with larva) and drinking areas (Mersha et al, 2012).

2.2.1.4. Anthropogenic/human factors

Construction of water schemes to meet the power and agricultural requirements for development have leads to increasing rates of transmission of schistosomiasis (Chitsulo*et al.*, 2000).

A major factor associated with the increase of schistosomiasis is water development projects,Particularly man-made lakes (hydroelectric power) and irrigation schemes (agriculture), which can lead to shiftsin snail vector populations (Patz*et al.*, 2000; WHO, 2002). On the other hand, water stagnation and weedgrowing due to inadequate water management sustain the life of the snails to complete the life cycle ofschistosomes (Boeele and Madsen, 2006).

Many surface irrigation systems in Africa create favorable snailbreedingconditions that facilitate the transmission of schistosomiasis (WHO, 2004). Irrigation schemes aredynamic agro-ecosystemsthat can transport snails a long way along the canals and where local events can eitherprovide habitat-friendly conditions or inhibit snail populations (Dale and Polasky, 2007).

2.2.2 Transmission

Schistosomes live in the mesenteric and hepatic veins of the host (except for S. nasale, which lives in the nasal veins), where they feed on blood and produce eggs with a characteristic terminal or lateral spine. Eggs passed in the feces must be deposited in water, hatch and release miracidia, which invade suitable water snails and develop through primary and secondary sporocysts to become cercariae (Fraser et al., 1991)

When fully mature,cercariae leave the snail and swim freely in the water, where they remain viable for several hours. Ruminants are usually infected with cercariae by penetration of the skin, although infection may be acquired orally while animals are drinking.

During penetration, cercariae develop into schistosomula, which are transported via the lymph and blood to ther predilection sites. The prepatent period varies according to the species but is generally 45–70 days (Kahn, 2011).

2.3 Pathogenesis

The pathogenesis of the schistosomiasis are caused by the eggs of the parasities and the immune responces of the host (Olivier *et al.*, 2004). The course of infection is often divided into three phases: migratory, acute and chronic. The migratory phase occurs when cercariae penetrate and migrate through the skin. This is often asymptomatic, but in sensitized patients, it may cause transient dermatitis ('swimmers itch'), and occasionally pulmonary lesions and pneumonitis (Olivier *et al.*, 2004).

Eggs released into the blood stream by adult worms can invade local tissues, where they release toxins and enzymes and provoke a TH-2-mediated immune response (Coutinho*et al.*, 2007). Inflammation and granuloma formation occurs around deposited eggs, which can lead to fibrosis and scarring of affected tissues, if the burden of eggs is heavy (Cheever *et al.*, 2000).

Eggs tend to either penetrate the bowel (adjacent to the mesenteric vessels in which the adult worms are residing) or travel via the portal venous system to the liver. In the bowel, granulomatous inflammation around the invading eggs can result in intestinal schistosomiasis characterized by ulceration and scarring (Friedman *et al.*, 2007)

2.4 Life Cycle

The adult females lay eggs in the capillaries of the intestinal wall. The egg masses form abscesses that finally burst and release the eggs into the gut, which are transported outside with the host's feces. Once outside and in contact with water the eggs release small swimming larvae, the miracidia, which find a suitable snail and penetrate into its body.

Inside the snail miracidia develop further during 1 to 4 months through two generations of sporocysts to asexually produce dozens of cercariae. Mature infective cercariae leave the snail through its respiratory hole. A single snail can release up to 3'000 cercariae(Kahn, 2011).

Parasite eggs are released into the environment from infected individuals, hatching on contact with fresh water to release the free-swimming miracidium. Miracidia infect freshwater snails by penetrating the snail's foot.

After infection, close to the site of penetration, the miracidium transforms into a primary (mother) sporocyst (Laurant, 2013).

Germ cells with in the primary sporocyst will then begin dividing to produce secondary (daughter) sporocysts, which migrate to the snail's hepatopancreas. Once at the hepatopancreas, germ cells with in the secondary sporocyst begin to divide again, this time producing thousands of new parasites, known as cercariae, which are the larvae capable of infecting mammals (Laurant, 2013).Cercariae emerge daily from the snail host in a circadian rhythm, dependent on ambient temperature and light.

Young cercariae are highly mobile, alternating between vigorous upward movements and sinking to maintain their position in the water.

Cercarial activity is particularly stimulated by water turbulence, by shadows and by chemicals found on human skin (Fenwick, 2012).Detailed schematic presentation of the life cycle of schestosomiasis is indicated in (Figure 2)

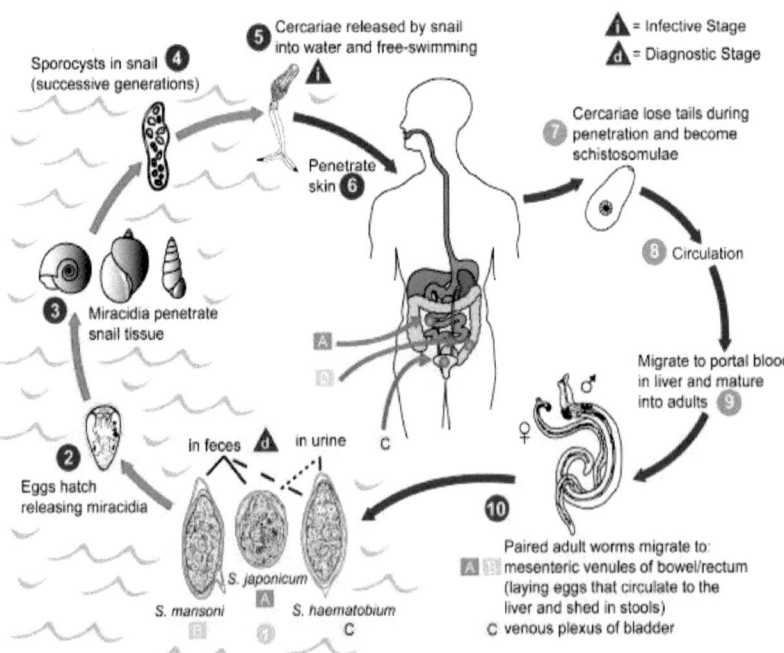

Figure 2: Life cycle of Schistosomes; Source: (CDC, 2011)

2.5 Clinical findings

The effects of schistosome infections of livestock are not easily recognized and the non-specific clinical signs are often overlooked by farmers. Infections may, however, result in severe clinical signs. The infections are often manifested by acute intestinal signs, 7-9weeks after infection the time when the females produce large numbers of eggs which penetrate the gut wall(Kahn, 2011).

The principal clinical signs are associated with passage of the spined eggs through the tissue of the gut lumen. In cattle the clinical sign exhibited emaciation marked diarrhea, mixed with blood or mucous, dehydration, pale of mucous membrane, marked weight loss, decreased production, rough hair coat, anemia, hypoalbuminemia, hyperglobulinemia and severe eosinophilia that develop after the onset of egg excretion. Severely affected animals deteriorate rapidly and usually die with in a few months of infection, while those less heavily infected develop chronic disease with growth retardation (Merck and Dhome, 2010).

Signs associated with chronic hepatic disease may develop when eggs are washed back to the liver by the portal circulation during their penetration of the gut wall. The eggs become lodged in the liver and an intense immunological response results, followed by the formation of a granuloma. A large proportion of the liver may be destroyed and the liver function severely disturbed (Mershaet al., 2012).

2.6 Diagnosis

For people from non-endemic areas or living in low transmission areas, serological and immunological tests may be useful in showing exposure to infection and the need for thorough examination and treatment. Urogenital Schistosomiasis can be diagnosed by filtration of urine followed by microscopic examination to detect *S. hematobium* eggs (Laikemariam,*et al,*2005). Serologic tests (e.g. Circumoval Precipitin test [CPT] and Indirect Hemaglutination Assay [IHA]) are improved tests for the detection of the presence of antibody against differet *Schistosoma* stages. Although these tests were found to be more sensitive, acute infection can not be distinguished from chronic infection.

Examination of stool and/or urine for ova is the primary methods of diagnosis for suspected schistosome infections. The choice of sample to diagnose schistosomiasis depends on the species of parasite likely causing the infection. Adult stages of S. mansoni, S. japonicum, S. mekongi, and S. intercalatum residein the mesenteric venous plexus of infected hosts and eggs are shed in feces; S. haematobium adult worms are found in the venous plexus of the lower urinary tract and eggs are shed in urine (CDC, 2012).

The routine methods used for parasitological diagnosis include; fecal smear, filtration method, sedimentation method, rectal and liver biopsy and miracidial hatching test. The most commonly used method for detection of fecal egg excretion under field condition is the sedimentation method (JalelNegero and BentiDeresa, 2017). At necropsy, *S. bovis* infection can be diagnosed by finding thousands of visible adult worms in the mesenteric veins. Infected livers are diagnosed on the basis of the presence of macroscopic lesions of schistosomiasis visible as white-gray foci under the liver capsule and with in the substance of the liver (Hendrix and Robinson, 2006).

2.7 Managements Of The Disease

2.7.1 Treatment

Infections with all major *Schistosoma species* can be treated with praziquantel. Treatment of schistosomiasis helps in reversing acute or early chronic disease, preventing complications associated with chronic infection and preventing neuro schistosomiasis. The goal of treatment is reduction of egg production via reduction of worm load: this reduces mortality and morbidity (Richer, 2003).Care has to be exercised in treating clinical cases of schistosomiasis since the dislodgement of the damaged flukes may result in emboli being formed and subsequent occlusion of major mesenteric and portal veins with fatal consequences (Urquhart *et al.*, 1996).

2.7.2 Control and prevention

The most effective way to control cattle schistosomiasis in endemic areas is to prevent contact between the animals and the parasite by fencing of dangerous waters and supplying clean water. Other methods of control include destruction of the snail intermediate host population at transmission sites, either by chemical or biological methods, or their removal by mechanical barriers or snail traps (Merck and Dohme, 2010). From the current available chemical Bayluscide (Niclosamide) and copper sulfate are the choices for molluscicide.

In addition to these, a native Ethiopia plant, *phytoplaca dodecandora*, locally known as "endod" is also an effective molluscicide (Shibru*et al.*, 1989).

Biological control of blood flukes (i.e. using their natural enemies) is so far not feasible.. Ecological measures against the snails that aim to render their habitat unsuitable for survival, such as drainage, removal of water weeds, and increased water flow, have also proved valuable. These measures not only help reduce the transmission of schistosomiasis but also help control other parasitic trematodes such as *Fasciola gigantica* and paramphistomes, which also have water snails as intermediate hosts and frequently are found in the same localities as schistosomes (Kahn, 2011). In human being, the most effective way of controlling Schistosomiasis are the provision of sanitary facilities and piped water since; it reduces human contact with contaminated water (Mohammad and Waqtola, 2006).

3. PREVALENCE OF THE DISEASE IN ETHIOPIA

In Ethiopia, the optimum range for distribution of S.mansoni has been reported as 1500 to 2000 meter above sea level (masl) (Gashaw, 2010). Detailed information on prevalence and intensity of infection of *S.bovis* in Ethiopia and various factors, which influence the host parasite relationship are generally lacking. However S. *bovis* has a localized distribution, which is found commonly in northern, eastern, southwestern and central parts of Ethiopia. The prevalence of bovine schistosomiasis was higher in local breed cattle (27.5%) than cross breed cattle(21.8%).

The highest prevalence of schistosoma infectionwas observed in cattle of 2 to 5 years of age (28.7%)followed by those older than 5 years while the lowest prevalence was observed in cattle of less than 2 years of age ((*Samuel et al, 2016*). Studies conducted in different parts of Ethiopia that reports different level of prevalence are summarized in table 2.

Table 2.Prevalence of Bovine schistosomiasis in different areas of Ethiopia

Author/s name	study area	prevalence reported
Lo andLemma (1973)	Awassa	5.5%
Solomon (1985)	Bahirdar	33%
Haile (1985)	Bahirdar	33%
Aemro (1993)	Bahirdar	12.3%
Hailu (1999)	Bahir Dar	34%
Ameni*et al.*, (2001)	Kamissie	28%
Yelelet., (2004)	Bahirdar	17.4%
Almaz (2007)	Bahirdar	10.93%
Solomon (2008)	Bahirdar	28.14%
Zelalem, (2010).	Fogera district	12.5%
Alemseged*et al.*, (2010)	Dembi district	27.13%
Mersha*et al .,(*2011)	South Gondar	13.7%
Abebe*et al.,(*2011)	Jimma Zone	13.46%
Mihrati andSamuel(2015)	DabireTabor	7.6%
Bereket*et al*(2015)	Damot woide district	81.3%
Addis,K.G(2017	Lalibela	25.9%
Abebu (2018)	Gewani	1.5%
Abebu (2018)	Awassa	5.5%
Abebe *et al*(2019)	South Achefer District	22.2%

4. ECONOMIC AND PUBILIC HEALTH SIGNIFICANCE OF THE DISEASE

4.1 Economic Importance

In attempting to estimate the economic importance of schistosomiasis one is strongly confronted with a varied array of factors for most of which there are no adequate measurements, among these factors are geographical distribution, prevalence, intensity of infection, clinical gradients, morbidity and mortality, and transmission patterns, which are influenced by environmental conditions, the relative efficiency of intermediate hosts and agricultural practices (Wright, 2015).

Although few or no overt clinical signs may be recognized in the short term, high prevalence rates of chronic schistosome infections cause significant losses on a herd basis. These losses are due to less easily recognizable effects on growth and productivity, as well as increased susceptibility to other parasitic and bacterial diseases (De Bont&Vercruysse, 1998).

According to (Cauleyet al., 1984) in addition to the high prevalence, outbreak of the disease and increased susceptibility to other parasitic and bacterial disease, the disease has an economic impact like production losses due to *S. bovis* that result from mortality, delayed growth, partial liver condemnation and poor future reproduction performance and sub-clinical infections cause significant losses due to long term effects on animal growth and productive capacity or milk yield and draft power.

4.2. Public Health Importance

Over 200 million people are infected over at least in 75 countries and 500 million peoples are exposed to infection. Schistosomiasis caused by *S. mansoni*, *S. haematobium* and *S. japonicum* is secondary only to malaria and affect approximately 200 million people in Africa, Asia, and South America (Bowman, 2003; Mohammad and Waqtola, 2006). Cercarial dermatitis or swimmer's itch is a condition caused when cercariae of blood flukes that normally parasitize aquatic birds and mammals penetrate the human skin, sensitizing the areas of attack and causing pustules and an itchy rash. Since humans are

17

not suitable definitive hosts for these flukes, the cercariae do not normally enter the blood stream and mature instead, after penetrating the skin, they are destroyed by the victim's immune response.

Allergenic material released from dead and dying cercariae produce a localized inflammatory reaction. Humans may become sensitized and develop pruritic macula papular, then vesicular skin lesions at the site of penetration. Skin lesions may be accompanied by a systemic febrile response that runs for 5 to 7 days and resolves spontaneously (Kahn, 2011)

Cercarial dermatitis occurs worldwide. In North America, ocean-related schistosome dermatitis (clam diggers itch) occurs on all Atlantic, Gulf, Pacific and Hawaiian coasts. It is common in muddy flats off Cape Cod. A form of cutaneous larvae migrants often called "swimmers itch" (cercarial dermatitis) occurs in man and Schistosomes which have a limited migration in human skin (Hendrix and Robinson, 2006) and it is common in some lakes regions. Humans serve as incidental hosts for these avian schistosomes. During the swimmer months, people swim or wade in the lakes, ponds, rivers and even ocean waters frequented by the wild birds.

5. CONCLUSION AND RECOMMENDATIONS

schistosomiasis is one of the endemic diseases of the animals and humans. which is caused by
species of schistosomes. *S. bovis*, the agent of schistosomiasis in cattle. It is one of the major veterinary problems in many Mediterranean and African countries. Occurrence of bovine
schistosomiasis is dependent on environmental factors such as moisture, rain fall, temperature, water bodies (stagnant, swampy and marshy) and snail intermediate hosts.
Few epidemiological studies conducted on bovine schistosomiasis in Ethiopia indicate, the endemicity of the disease in the country. Although few or no overt clinical signs may

18

be recognized in case of bovine schistosomiasis in the short term, high prevalence of chronic schistosome infections cause significant losses on a herd basis. Therefore, it is important to obtain more information on natural schistosome's infection in cattle in general, and on the evaluation of the host–parasite relationship under condition of challenge in particular.

The economic significance of the disease is mainly attributed to morbidity, mortality, liver condemnation, reduced productivity and poor subsequent reproductive performance. However,still there a limitation on detailed information of epidemiology; and various factors, which influence the host parasite relationship, prevention and control strategies.

Based on the above conclusion, the following recommendations are given

> In endemic areas, public awareness is important to avoid swimming in potentially infested water bodies and to protect their livestock in high risk areas.

> Human being after swimming must be washed the bodies with soap and dry with clean towel.

> Detailed study on the epidemiology of the disease like malacological and parasitological survey, and mapping high risk areas should be carried out for sound prevention and control of schistosomiasis.

> Available means in snail control and disease monitoring could be implemented as a short term activity.

> The native Ethiopian plant *phytoplancca dodecandora*, locally known as "Endod" which is considered as potent molluscicide for the control of human Schistosomosis, could also be effectively used against intermediate host of *S. bovis*.

6. REFERENCES

Abebe, F., Behablom, M. and Berhanu, M. (2011). Major Trematode Infections of Cattle Slaughtered at Jimma Municipal Abattoir and the Occurrence of intermediate hosts in Selected Water Bodies of the Zone. *Journal of Animal and Veterinary Advances; 10(12): 1592-1597*

Abebe,Y., Befikadu,U., and Getachew,A.(2019). Prevalence and risk factors of bovine schistosomiasis in Northwestern Ethiopia. *BMC Veterinary Research;15:12*.https://doi.org/10.1186/s12917-018-1757-9

Abebu,W.,(2018).A Study on Prevalence of Bovine Schistosomiasis in Fogera Woreda North Western of Ethiopi.

Addis,K.G.(2017). Prevalence and Associated Risk Factors of Bovine Schistosomiasis in Northwestern Ethiopia. *World's Veterinary Journa*; l7(1):pp 01-04

Aemro, T. (1993) Assessment of prevalence, economic significance and drug efficacy trial on bovine Schistosomosis in Bahir Dar, Ethiopia. DVM Thesis, faculty of veterinary medicine, Addis Ababa University, DebreZeit, Ethiopi;.**23**:76-78.

Alemseged, G., (2010). Prevalence of bovine schistosomiasis in Dembia District North west Ethiopia.Dvm thesis, faculty of veterinary medicine. Gondar, Ethiopia.

Ameni, G., Krok, B. and Bogale, T. (2001).Preliminary study on the major bovine trematode infection around Kemissie, Northeastern Ethiopia and treatment trial with praziquantel. *Bull Animal. Heath. Production. Africa,* **49**: 62-67

Bedarkar, S.N., Narladkar, B.W. and Deshpande, P.D. (2000). Seasonal prevalence of snail fluke infections in ruminants of Marathwada region.*Journal of Veterinary Parasitology;* **14**(1): 51-54.

Belayneh L and Tadesse G (2014). Bovine schistosomiasis:a threat in public health perspective in Bahirdar town, North West Ethiopia. *Acta parasitological Globalis,* **5** (1): 01-06.

Belayneh, L. and G. Tadesse, (2012). Bovine schistosomiasis: A Threat in Public Health perspective in Bahir Dar Town, Northwest Ethiopia.*Acta Parasitological Globalis; 5(1): 1-6.*

Bereket,A . and Zewudneh,T.(2015). Schistosoma mansoni infection prevalence and associated risk factors among schoolchildren in Demba Girara, Damot Woide District of Wolaita Zone, Southern Ethiopia. *Asian Pacific Journal of Tropical Medicine;8(6):457-463*

Boelee. E. Madsen, H. (2006). Irrigation and schistosomiasis in Africa: Ecological aspects. Colombo, Sri Lanka: *International Water Management Institute. IWMI Research Report 99:39.*

Bon,t J.D. (1995). *Cattle Schistosomosis*: host parasite interactions. PhD. Thesis, University of Gent, **23.**

Bont JD. (1997). *Cattle Schistosomosis*: host parasite interactions. PhD. Thesis, University of Gent, 23.

Bushara, H.O, Hussein, M.F., Majid, M.A., Taylor, M.G.(1982) Effectives of praziquantel and metrifonate on Schistosomabovis.*American Journal of Tropical Medicine and Hygiene; 29: 442-451.*

Cheever. AW, Hoffmann. KF, Wynn. TA. (2000) Immuno pathology of schistosomiasis mansoni in mice and men.Chemotherapy.Angewandte Chemie (International ed. in English) **52**: 7936–7956.

Coutinho.H.M, Acosta. L.P., Wu. H.W. (2007) Th2 cytokines are associated with persistent hepatic fibrosis in human Schistosoma japonicum infection. *J Infect Dis* **195**:288.

Dale, V.H,and Polasky ,S (2007).Measures of the effects of agricultural practices on ecosystem services. *Ecol. Econ.* **64**:286-296.

Dargie, J.D.(1980). The pathogenesis of schistosoma bovis infection in Sudanese cattle.*Foy.Soc.Trop.Med.Hyg.*,**74**: 560-562.

De Bont J &Vercruysse, J. (1998) Schistosomiasis in cattle.*AdvParasitology* . **41**: 286–364

De Bont, J.and Vercruysse,J. (1999) The epidemiology and control of cattle schistosomiasis. *Parasitol.Today:* **13**:255-262.

Fraser, C.M., Bergeron, J.A., Maya, A. and Susan, E.A. (1991). The Merck veterinary manual: A handbook of diagnosis, therapy, and disease prevention and control for the veterinarian, 7th edition U.S.A, *Merck and Co., Inc. Pp 76-78.*

Friedman.J.F, Mital. P, Kanzaria. H.K (2007) Schistosomiasis and pregnancy. *Trends Parasitol 23: 159*

Gabriel, S., De Bont, I.K., Phiri, M., Masuku, G., Riveau, A.M., Schacht, A.M., Deelder, G., and J. Vercruysse (2002). Transplacental transfer of schistosomal circulating anodic antigens in calves. *Parasite Immunology*, **24**: 521-525.

Gashaw.A (2010). Epidemiology of intestinal schistosoma in Hayk town, North East Ethiopia. Addis Ababa.

Haile, A. (1985). Observations on the prevalence of Schistosoma bovis infection in Bahir Dar area, North Central Ethiopia.DVM Thesis, faulty of Veterinary Medicine, Addis Ababa University, DebreZeit, Ethiopia.

Hailu, M., (1999). Observations on the prevalence and intensity of *Schistosoma bovis* infection in Bahir Dar area, north central Ethiopia. DVM Thesis, Faculty of Veterinary Medicine, Addis Ababa University.

Hendrix, M.C and Robinson, D.E (2006). Diagnostic Parasitology for Veterinary Technicians, 3[rd]ed. *New York: Academic press.*

Houdijk, J.G.M. and Athana, S.S.A.(2003). Direct and indirect effects of host nutrition on ruminants gastro intestinal parasites. *In:* Proceedings of the sixth International symposium on the nutrition of herbivores. Merida Mexico.

Ibrahim, M.Y.A., (2009). Studies on Molluscicidal Activity of Some Plants from Darfuragainst B truncates with Emphasis on Alternantheranodiflora (Amaranthaceae).PhD. Thesis, University of Khartoum.

Islam, M. N., Begum, N., Alam,A. Z. and. Mamun, M. A. A. (2000) Epidemiology of intestinal Schistosomiasis in ruminants of Bangladesh. J. Bangladesh Agril. Univ. 6 Marquardt.C.R, Greive B.R. Parasitology and vector biology. 2nd ed. Sandiago: Harcourt acadamic press Pp 265-272. *Journal of Veterinary Science & Medicine.* Volume **6** Issue 2.

Kahn, C.M ,(2011). The Merck veterinary manual. 10th ed. *White-house Station, NJ: Merck. & Co., Inc; pp. 273–1036.*

Kassew, A., (2007). Major Animal Health problems of marketing oriented livestock Development in Fogera woreda. DVM Thesis, Addis Ababa University, Faculty of Veterinary Medicine.Debere-Zeit, Ethiopia.

Kassi, T. (1999). Veterinary helminthology, 1st ed. England. *Butter worth Heinemann,* pp: 18-220

Laikemariam, K.O., Anteneh, T., Wutet, T., Tadele,K., Fekadu and AbdiBeker, (2005). Schistosomiasis Diploma program for the Ethiopian health center Module pp: 1-81.

Laurent.S.A, Boissier,J,and Robert.A,etal. (2013) Schistosomiasis

Liang, S., E. Seto, J. Remais, B. Zhong, Y. Yang, G. Davis, X. Gu, D. Qiu and R. Spear, (2007). Environmental effects on parasitic disease transmission exemplified by schistosomiasis in western China. *USA, Proc. Natl. Acad. Sci.,* **104:** 7110-7115.

LO and Lemma, A..A., (1973). Study on Schistosoma bovis.Annals of Tropical Medicine and Parasitology, **69** (3): 375-382.

Magona, J.W. and Musisi, G.(2002). Influence of age, grazing system, season and agro climatic zone on the prevalence and intensity of gastro intestinal strongylosis in Ugandan goats. *Small Ruminants Research,* **44**: 187-192.

Mandal. C.S (2012) Veterinary parasitology, 2nd ed. Kushnuma complex Basement, Ib Dwight, D., G. Bowman and M. Georgis, (2003).Parasitological for veterinarians. Elsevier (USA),

Mandal.C.S (2012). Veterinary parasitology, 2nd ed. *Kushnuma complex Basement, Ibdc publisher Pp 42-70.*

Marquardt. C.R, Greive B.R (2000) Parasitology and vector biology. 2nd ed. *Sandiago*: *Harcourt acadamic press* Pp 265-272.

Mersha, C., D. Belay and F. Tewodros, (2012). Prevalence of Cattle Schistosomiasis and Associated Risk Factors in Fogera Cattle, South Gondar Zone Amhara National Regional State, Ethiopia. *Journal of Advanced Veterinary Research,* **2:** 153-156.

Mohammad A.A. Waqtola, C. (2006). *Medical Parasitology Jimma University*, Ethiopia, USAID. pp. 284-300.

Nagi, M.A.N., A. Kumar, J.S. Mubara and S.A. Mashmoos, (1999).Epidemiology, Clinical and Haematological profile of Schistosomiasis. *American Eurasian Journal of Scientific Research;* **4**(1): 14-19.

Oliveira, G., Rodrigues, N.B. and Romanha,A.J *et al*. (2004). Genome and Genomics of Schistosomes. *Canadian Journal of zoology*, **82**(2):375-390.

Parija. CS (2004) Text book of Parasitology, protozology and helminthology. 2nd ed. Chennai: AIPD. p. 141-256.

Patz, J., Graczyk, T., Gelle,r N and Vitor, A.Y (2000). Effects of environmental change on emerging parasite diseases.*International Journal of Parasitology;***30:**1395-405.

Richer (2003); the impact of chemotherapy on morbidity due to schistosomiasis.*Acta trop*: **86** (2-3): 161

Samuel. A, Sefinew,A. Samuel . D, Yitayew.D, and Dagmawi ,Y.(2016).A CrossSectional Study on the Prevalence and Possible Risk Factors of Bovine Schistosomiasis in and Around Bahir Dar Town, Northwest Ethiopia.*European Journal of Biological Sciences* **8** (1): 14-20.

Shibru T, Getachew T, Hailu B. *Parasitology*. Ins. Shibru T., Getachew, T. and Kloos, H. (1989).Schistosomosis in Ethiopia. *Addis Ababa: Addis Ababa Printing press, pp. 18 - 26.*

Solomon, H. (1985).*Schistosomosis in domestic ruminants in BahirDar*.DVM thesis, FVM, AAU, DebreZeit. Ethiopia.

Urquhart, G.M., Armour, J., Duncan, J.L., Dunn, A.M. and Jennings, F.W (2003). Veterinary Parasitology. 2nd ed. Scotland: Black well science,pp 117-120.

Urquhart, G.M.; Armour, J.; Duncan J.L. and Jenning, F.W. (1996). Veterinary helminthology veterinary parasitology *New York Churchill Livingstone Inc*. pp. 117-119

Vercruysse, J.and Gabriel S.(2005). Parasite Immunology. Volume **27:** pages 289–295

WHO, (2010). Schistosomiasis: Population requiring preventive chemotherapy and number of people treated in, *Wkly Epidemiology*, **87**: 37-44.

Woldemichael, T., D. Asfaw, A. Dawit, T. Geremew, M. Yared, T. Frehiwot and M. Daniel, (2006). Screening of some medicinal plants of Ethiopia for their molluscicidal activities and phytochemical constituents. *Pharmacology Online*; **3**: 245-258.

World Health Organization (WHO) (2002).Prevention and control of schistosomiasis and soil-transmitted helminthiasis, WHO technical report series, Geneva.

World Health Organization (WHO) (2004). WHO: Prevention and Control of Schistosomiasis and Soil-Transmitted Helminthiasis. WHO Technical Report Series, Geneva.

Wrigh,t W. H.(2015). A consideration of the economic impact of schistosomiasis.Bull World Health .

Zelalem, A., (2010). Prevalence of bovine schistosomiasis in FogeraWoredaBussiness paper Submitted to Faculty of Veterinary Medicine, University of Gondar. **82**: 375–390.

YOUR KNOWLEDGE HAS VALUE

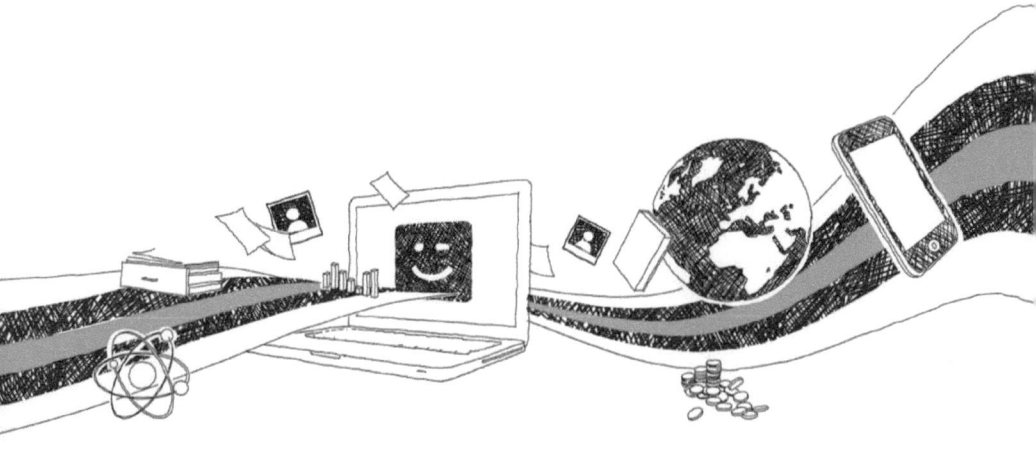

- We will publish your bachelor's and
  master's thesis, essays and papers

- Your own eBook and book -
  sold worldwide in all relevant shops

- Earn money with each sale

Upload your text at www.GRIN.com
and publish for free

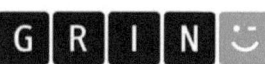